I0757054

THE OSTEOPOROSIS DIET COOKBOOK

20 Nourishing Recipes for Strong Bones

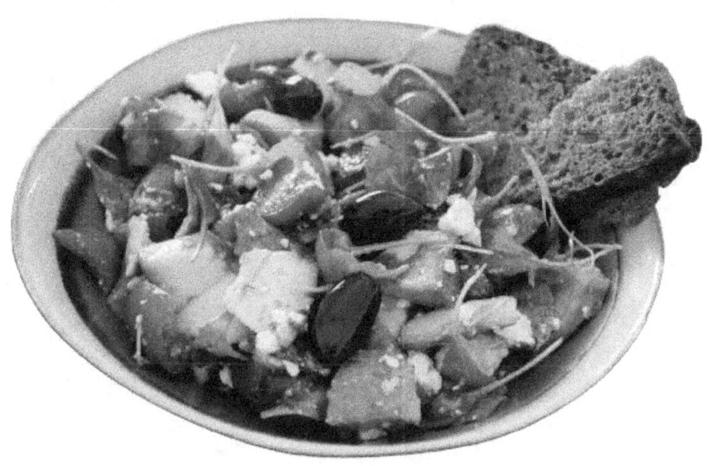

Willie S. Harper

Copyright © 2023, Willie S. Harper

All rights reserved. No part of this book may be reproduced, stored in a retrieval system, or transmitted in any form or by any means, electronic, mechanical, photocopying, recording, scanning, or otherwise, without the prior written permission of the copyright holder. This book is sold subject to the condition that it shall not, by way of trade or otherwise, be lent, resold, hired out or otherwise circulated without the prior consent of the copyright holder in any form of binding or cover other than that in which it is published and without a similar condition including this condition being imposed on the subsequent purchaser

OTHER BOOKS BY THE AUTHOR

HASHIMOTO DIET FOR NEWLY DIAGNOSED RECIPE COOKBOOK

NO GALLBLADDER DIET RECIPE COOKBOOK

INSULIN RESISTANCE DIET COOKBOOK

PLANT BASED MEDITERRANEAN DIET COOKBOOK

JUICING FOR CANCER RECIPE BOOK FOR NEWLY DIAGNOSED

JUICING FOR DIABETES RECIPE BOOK

ALZHEIMER'S SOLUTION DIET COOKBOOK FOR BEGINNERS

DIVERTICULITIS DIET COOKBOOK

ACID REFLUX DIET COOKBOOK FOR BEGINNERS

AYURVEDA COOKBOOK FOR WOMEN

LOW OXALATE DIET BOOK

BARIATRIC DIET COOKBOOK

JUICING RECIPES FOR GUT HEALTH

AFIB COOKBOOK

THE AUTOIMMUNE PROTOCOL COOKBOOK

HEART HEALTHY COOKBOOK FOR BEGINNERS 2023

GOUT DIET COOKBOOK

RENAL DIET SMOOTHIE RECIPES FOR SENIORS

DIABETIC RENAL DIET COOKBOOKCIRRHOSIS DIET CONTROL COOKBOOK

TABLE OF CONTENT

INTRODUCTION

Emily was determined to strengthen her fragile bones and stop the osteoporosis-related bone loss that was already happening. Emily used to reside in a little hamlet. Her aggravation with the lack of knowledge led her to find "The Osteoporosis Diet Cookbook: 20 Nourishing Recipes for Strong Bones."

Curiosity drove Emily to swiftly delve into its pages, where she found a wealth of knowledge and recipes. As she started her culinary profession, she discovered the importance of a nutrient-rich diet in enhancing bone health. Each meal offered a delicious and inventive way to eat healthy, from delectable salmon dinners to calcium-boosting smoothie bowls. With each bite, Emily felt a burst of energy and vibrancy.

Along with delicious meals, the book gave her advice on healthy living, necessary minerals, and exercises for strong bones. Emily learned as her journey progressed that this book served as her guide to a healthier, osteoporosis-free future.

Chapter 1: Breakfast Delights: Starting the Day with Bone-Nourishing Recipes

Calcium-Boosting Smoothie Bowl

- 1 frozen banana
- 1 cup spinach
- ½ cup Greek yogurt
- ¼ cup almond milk
- 1 tablespoon chia seeds
- 2 tablespoons almond butter
- Toppings: sliced strawberries, blueberries, granola

Instructions:

1. In a blender, combine the frozen banana, spinach, Greek yogurt, almond milk, chia seeds, and almond butter.
2. Blend until smooth and creamy.
3. Pour the smoothie mixture into a bowl.
4. Top with sliced strawberries, blueberries, and granola.
5. Serve immediately.

Serving: 1 bowl

Cook time: 5 minutes

Nutritional Information per Serving: Calories: 380, Protein: 15g, Fat: 18g, Carbohydrates: 45g, Fiber: 9g

Veggie Omelet with Spinach and Feta

- 2 large eggs
- ¼ cup chopped spinach
- 2 tablespoons crumbled feta cheese
- 1 tablespoon chopped fresh herbs (such as parsley or dill)
- Salt and pepper to taste
- Cooking spray

Instructions:

1. In a bowl, whisk the eggs until well beaten.
2. Stir in the chopped spinach, crumbled feta cheese, chopped herbs, salt, and pepper.
3. Heat a non-stick skillet over medium heat and coat it with cooking spray.
4. Pour the egg mixture into the skillet and cook for 2-3 minutes, or until the edges start to set.
5. Flip the omelet and cook for an additional 1-2 minutes, or until the eggs are fully cooked.
6. Slide the omelet onto a plate and fold it in half.
7. Serve hot.

Serving: 1 omelet

Cook time: 10 minutes

Nutritional Information per Serving: Calories: 210, Protein: 18g, Fat: 14g, Carbohydrates: 2g, Fiber: 1g

Overnight Chia Seed Pudding with Berries

- ¼ cup chia seeds
- 1 cup almond milk
- 1 tablespoon maple syrup
- ½ teaspoon vanilla extract
- Fresh berries for topping

Instructions:

1. In a bowl or jar, combine the chia seeds, almond milk, maple syrup, and vanilla extract.
2. Stir well to combine all the ingredients.
3. Cover the bowl or jar and refrigerate overnight or for at least 4 hours.
4. Stir the mixture once or twice during the chilling time to prevent clumping.
5. Before serving, give the pudding a good stir to ensure a smooth consistency.
6. Top with fresh berries.
7. Enjoy chilled.

Serving: 1 bowl

Cook time: 4 hours (includes chilling time)

Nutritional Information per Serving: Calories: 220, Protein: 8g, Fat: 11g, Carbohydrates: 23g, Fiber: 13g

Whole Grain Pancakes with Greek Yogurt Topping

- 1 cup whole wheat flour
- 1 tablespoon baking powder
- 1 tablespoon honey
- 1 cup almond milk
- 1 large egg
- Cooking spray
- Greek yogurt and fresh fruit for topping

Instructions:

1. In a bowl, whisk together the whole wheat flour and baking powder.
2. In a separate bowl, beat the honey, almond milk, and egg until well combined.
3. Pour the wet ingredients into the dry ingredients and stir until just combined. Do not overmix; lumps are okay.
4. Heat a non-stick skillet or griddle over medium heat and coat it with cooking spray.
5. Pour ¼ cup of batter onto the skillet for each pancake.
6. Cook for 2-3 minutes, or until bubbles form on the surface.
7. Flip the pancakes and cook for an additional 1-2 minutes, or until golden brown.
8. Serve the pancakes topped with Greek yogurt and fresh fruit.

Serving: 2 pancakes

Cook time: 15 minutes

Nutritional Information per Serving: Calories: 250, Protein: 10g, Fat: 4g, Carbohydrates: 46g, Fiber: 6g

Chapter 2: Wholesome Lunches: Satisfying Meals for Bone Health

Superfood Salad with Kale, Quinoa, and Avocado

- 2 cups chopped kale
- 1 cup cooked quinoa
- ½ avocado, diced
- ¼ cup dried cranberries
- ¼ cup chopped walnuts
- 2 tablespoons lemon juice
- 1 tablespoon olive oil
- Salt and pepper to taste

Instructions:

1. In a large bowl, combine the chopped kale, cooked quinoa, diced avocado, dried cranberries, and chopped walnuts.
2. In a small bowl, whisk together the lemon juice, olive oil, salt, and pepper to make the dressing.
3. Drizzle the dressing over the salad and toss to coat all the ingredients.
4. Serve immediately or refrigerate until ready to eat.

Serving: 2 servings

Preparation time: 15 minutes

Nutritional Information per Serving: Calories: 350, Protein: 10g, Fat: 20g, Carbohydrates: 40g, Fiber: 8g

Salmon and Broccoli Stir-Fry

- 2 salmon fillets, skinless and boneless
- 2 cups broccoli florets
- 1 red bell pepper, sliced
- 2 cloves garlic, minced
- 2 tablespoons low-sodium soy sauce
- 1 tablespoon honey
- 1 tablespoon sesame oil
- 1 tablespoon cornstarch
- ¼ cup water
- Sesame seeds for garnish (optional)

Instructions:

1. Cut the salmon fillets into bite-sized pieces.
2. In a small bowl, whisk together the soy sauce, honey, sesame oil, cornstarch, and water to make the sauce.
3. Heat a large skillet or wok over medium-high heat and add a little oil.
4. Add the minced garlic and cook for 1 minute until fragrant.
5. Add the salmon pieces to the skillet and cook for 3-4 minutes until lightly browned.
6. Add the broccoli florets and red bell pepper slices to the skillet and stir-fry for an additional 4-5 minutes until the vegetables are tender-crisp.
7. Pour the sauce over the salmon and vegetables and stir well to coat everything.
8. Continue cooking for 2-3 minutes until the sauce thickens.

9. Sprinkle with sesame seeds, if desired, and serve hot.

Serving: 2 servings

Preparation time: 20 minutes

Nutritional Information per Serving: Calories: 400, Protein: 30g, Fat: 18g, Carbohydrates: 30g, Fiber: 6g

Lentil Soup with Leafy Greens

- 1 cup dried green lentils, rinsed and drained
- 1 onion, chopped
- 2 carrots, diced
- 2 stalks celery, diced
- 3 cloves garlic, minced
- 4 cups vegetable broth
- 2 cups water
- 2 cups chopped leafy greens (such as spinach or kale)
- 1 teaspoon cumin
- 1 teaspoon paprika
- Salt and pepper to taste
- Fresh lemon juice for garnish

Instructions:

1. In a large pot, heat a little oil over medium heat.
2. Add the chopped onion, carrots, celery, and minced garlic. Sauté for 5 minutes until the vegetables are softened.

3. Add the rinsed lentils, vegetable broth, water, cumin, paprika, salt, and pepper to the pot.
4. Bring the mixture to a boil, then reduce the heat to low, cover, and simmer for 20-25 minutes until the lentils are tender.
5. Stir in the chopped leafy greens and cook for an additional 5 minutes until wilted.
6. Taste and adjust the seasoning if needed.
7. Serve the soup hot, squeezing fresh lemon juice over each bowl for added flavor.

Serving: 4 servings

Preparation time: 35 minutes

Nutritional Information per Serving: Calories: 250, Protein: 15g, Fat: 1g, Carbohydrates: 45g, Fiber: 15g

Greek-Style Stuffed Peppers

- 2 bell peppers (any color), halved and seeded
- 1 cup cooked quinoa
- ½ cup crumbled feta cheese
- ¼ cup chopped Kalamata olives
- 2 tablespoons chopped fresh parsley
- 1 tablespoon lemon juice
- 1 tablespoon olive oil
- Salt and pepper to taste

Instructions:

1. Preheat the oven to 375°F (190°C).
2. In a bowl, combine the cooked quinoa, crumbled feta cheese, chopped Kalamata olives, chopped fresh parsley, lemon juice, olive oil, salt, and pepper.
3. Stuff the halved bell peppers with the quinoa mixture, pressing it down gently.
4. Place the stuffed peppers on a baking sheet and bake in the preheated oven for 25-30 minutes until the peppers are tender and the filling is heated through.
5. Remove from the oven and let them cool for a few minutes before serving.

Serving: 2 servings

Preparation time: 35 minutes

Nutritional Information per Serving: Calories: 300, Protein: 10g, Fat: 12g, Carbohydrates: 40g, Fiber: 8g

Chapter 3: Nourishing Dinners: Flavorful Recipes for Strong Bones

Baked Salmon with Lemon and Dill

- 2 salmon fillets
- 2 tablespoons fresh lemon juice
- 1 tablespoon olive oil
- 1 tablespoon chopped fresh dill
- Salt and pepper to taste
- Lemon slices for garnish

Instructions:

1. Preheat the oven to 375°F (190°C) and line a baking sheet with parchment paper.
2. Place the salmon fillets on the prepared baking sheet.
3. In a small bowl, whisk together the lemon juice, olive oil, chopped dill, salt, and pepper.
4. Pour the lemon-dill mixture over the salmon fillets, making sure they are evenly coated.
5. Place a few lemon slices on top of each fillet.
6. Bake in the preheated oven for 12-15 minutes, or until the salmon is cooked through and flakes easily with a fork.
7. Remove from the oven and let it rest for a few minutes before serving.

Serving: 2 servings

Preparation time: 20 minutes

Nutritional Information per Serving: Calories: 300, Protein: 30g, Fat: 18g, Carbohydrates: 2g, Fiber: 0g

Spinach and Mushroom Stuffed Chicken Breast

- 2 boneless, skinless chicken breasts
- 1 cup chopped spinach
- ½ cup sliced mushrooms
- 2 cloves garlic, minced
- ¼ cup shredded mozzarella cheese
- 1 tablespoon olive oil
- Salt and pepper to taste

Instructions:

1. Preheat the oven to 400°F (200°C) and line a baking dish with parchment paper.
2. In a skillet, heat the olive oil over medium heat.
3. Add the minced garlic and sauté for 1 minute until fragrant.
4. Add the chopped spinach and sliced mushrooms to the skillet. Cook until the vegetables are wilted and any excess liquid has evaporated.
5. Remove the skillet from the heat and stir in the shredded mozzarella cheese. Let the mixture cool slightly.
6. Cut a pocket horizontally in each chicken breast, being careful not to cut all the way through.

7. Stuff each chicken breast with the spinach and mushroom mixture, pressing the edges together to seal the pocket.
8. Place the stuffed chicken breasts in the prepared baking dish and season with salt and pepper.
9. Bake in the preheated oven for 20-25 minutes or until the chicken is cooked through and no longer pink in the center.
10. Let the chicken rest for a few minutes before slicing and serving.

Serving: 2 servings

Preparation time: 30 minutes

Nutritional Information per Serving: Calories: 300, Protein: 40g, Fat: 12g, Carbohydrates: 4g, Fiber: 2g

Quinoa-Stuffed Bell Peppers

- 2 bell peppers (any color), tops removed and seeds removed
- ½ cup cooked quinoa
- ¼ cup black beans, rinsed and drained
- ¼ cup corn kernels
- ¼ cup diced tomatoes
- 2 tablespoons chopped fresh cilantro
- 1 tablespoon lime juice
- 1 teaspoon cumin
- Salt and pepper to taste

- Shredded cheddar cheese for topping (optional)

Instructions:

1. Preheat the oven to 375°F (190°C) and grease a baking dish.
2. In a bowl, combine the cooked quinoa, black beans, corn kernels, diced tomatoes,chopped cilantro, lime juice, cumin, salt, and pepper.
3. Stuff the bell peppers with the quinoa mixture, pressing it down gently. Top with shredded cheddar cheese if desired.
4. Place the stuffed bell peppers in the prepared baking dish.
5. Bake in the preheated oven for 25-30 minutes, or until the peppers are tender and the filling is heated through.
6. Remove from the oven and let them cool for a few minutes before serving.

Serving: 2 servings

Preparation time: 40 minutes

Nutritional Information per Serving: Calories: 250, Protein: 10g, Fat: 5g, Carbohydrates: 45g, Fiber: 8g

Lentil and Vegetable Curry

- 1 cup dried red lentils, rinsed and drained
- 1 onion, chopped
- 2 carrots, diced

- 1 bell pepper, diced
- 2 cloves garlic, minced
- 1 tablespoon curry powder
- 1 teaspoon ground cumin
- 1 teaspoon ground coriander
- ½ teaspoon turmeric
- ¼ teaspoon cayenne pepper (optional, adjust to taste)
- 2 cups vegetable broth
- 1 cup coconut milk
- 2 tablespoons tomato paste
- Salt and pepper to taste
- Fresh cilantro for garnish

Instructions:

1. In a large pot, heat a little oil over medium heat.
2. Add the chopped onion, diced carrots, diced bell pepper, and minced garlic. Sauté for 5 minutes until the vegetables are softened.
3. Stir in the curry powder, cumin, coriander, turmeric, and cayenne pepper. Cook for 1 minute until fragrant.
4. Add the rinsed lentils, vegetable broth, coconut milk, and tomato paste to the pot. Stir well to combine.
5. Bring the mixture to a boil, then reduce the heat to low. Cover and simmer for 20-25 minutes, or until the lentils are tender and the flavors have melded together.
6. Season with salt and pepper to taste.
7. Serve the lentil curry hot, garnished with fresh cilantro.

Serving: 4 servings

Preparation time: 40 minutes

Nutritional Information per Serving: Calories: 350, Protein: 15g, Fat: 15g, Carbohydrates: 45g, Fiber: 12g

Chapter 4: Wholesome Snacks and Treats: Delicious Bites for Bone Health

Almond Butter and Banana Toast

- 2 slices whole-grain bread
- 2 tablespoons almond butter
- 1 ripe banana, sliced
- 1 teaspoon honey (optional)

Instructions:

1. Toast the slices of whole-grain bread until golden and crisp.
2. Spread almond butter evenly on each slice.
3. Arrange the banana slices on top of the almond butter.
4. Drizzle with honey, if desired.
5. Serve the almond butter and banana toast as a nutritious snack or light breakfast option.

Serving: 1 serving

Preparation time: 5 minutes

Nutritional Information per Serving: Calories: 300, Protein: 8g, Fat: 12g, Carbohydrates: 45g, Fiber: 8g

Greek Yogurt Parfait with Berries and Granola

- 1 cup Greek yogurt
- ½ cup mixed berries (such as strawberries, blueberries, and raspberries)
- ¼ cup granola
- 1 tablespoon honey

Instructions:

1. In a glass or bowl, layer Greek yogurt, mixed berries, and granola.
2. Drizzle with honey.
3. Repeat the layers until all the ingredients are used.
4. Serve the Greek yogurt parfait as a satisfying and nutrient-rich snack or dessert.

Serving: 1 serving

Preparation time: 5 minutes

Nutritional Information per Serving: Calories: 250, Protein: 15g, Fat: 6g, Carbohydrates: 35g, Fiber: 6g

Roasted Chickpeas

- 1 can chickpeas, rinsed and drained
- 1 tablespoon olive oil
- 1 teaspoon paprika
- ½ teaspoon garlic powder
- ½ teaspoon cumin
- ¼ teaspoon cayenne pepper (optional, adjust to taste)

- Salt to taste

Instructions:

1. Preheat the oven to 400°F (200°C) and line a baking sheet with parchment paper.
2. In a bowl, toss the rinsed and drained chickpeas with olive oil, paprika, garlic powder, cumin, cayenne pepper (if using), and salt.
3. Spread the seasoned chickpeas in a single layer on the prepared baking sheet.
4. Roast in the preheated oven for 25-30 minutes, shaking the pan occasionally, until the chickpeas are crispy and golden.
5. Remove from the oven and let them cool before enjoying as a crunchy and protein-packed snack.

Serving: 2 servings

Preparation time: 35 minutes

Nutritional Information per Serving: Calories: 200, Protein: 10g, Fat: 6g, Carbohydrates: 30g, Fiber: 8g

Dark Chocolate and Almond Energy Balls

- 1 cup pitted dates
- ½ cup almonds
- ¼ cup dark chocolate chips
- 2 tablespoons cocoa powder
- 1 tablespoon almond butter

- 1 tablespoon honey
- 1 teaspoon vanilla extract
- Pinch of salt
- Shredded coconut for rolling (optional)

Instructions:

1. Place the pitted dates, almonds, dark chocolate chips, cocoa powder, almond butter, honey, vanilla extract, and salt in a food processor.
2. Process the mixture until well combined and the ingredients stick together.
3. Roll the mixture into small balls, about 1 inch in diameter.
4. If desired, roll the energy balls in shredded coconut for added flavor and texture.
5. Place the energy balls in an airtight container and refrigerate for at least 1 hour before serving.
6. Enjoy the dark chocolate and almond energy balls as a healthy and satisfying snack.

Serving: Approximately 12 energy balls

Preparation time: 15 minutes

Nutritional Information per Serving (1 energy ball): Calories: 120, Protein: 2g, Fat: 6g, Carbohydrates: 16g, Fiber: 3g

Chapter 6: Refreshing Beverages: Hydrating Drinks for Strong Bones

Green Smoothie

- 1 cup fresh spinach leaves
- 1 ripe banana
- ½ cup chopped cucumber
- ½ cup sliced pineapple
- 1 tablespoon chia seeds
- 1 cup almond milk (or any milk of your choice)
- Ice cubes (optional)

Instructions:

1. In a blender, combine the fresh spinach leaves, ripe banana, chopped cucumber, sliced pineapple, chia seeds, and almond milk.
2. Blend until smooth and creamy.
3. If desired, add ice cubes to make the smoothie colder and more refreshing.
4. Pour the green smoothie into a glass and enjoy as a nutrient-packed beverage.

Serving: 1 serving

Preparation time: 5 minutes

Nutritional Information per Serving: Calories: 200, Protein: 5g, Fat: 7g, Carbohydrates: 35g, Fiber: 9g

Berry Infused Water

- 1 cup mixed berries (such as strawberries, blueberries, and raspberries)
- 2 cups water
- Ice cubes

Instructions:

1. In a pitcher, add the mixed berries.
2. Pour the water over the berries and stir gently.
3. Place the pitcher in the refrigerator and let the berries infuse the water for at least 1 hour.
4. When ready to serve, add ice cubes to the glasses and pour the berry-infused water.
5. Enjoy the refreshing and hydrating berry-infused water as a healthy alternative to sugary drinks.

Serving: 2 servings

Preparation time: 5 minutes (plus infusion time)

Nutritional Information per Serving: Calories: 20, Protein: 0g, Fat: 0g, Carbohydrates: 5g, Fiber: 2g

Turmeric Ginger Tea

- 1 cup water
- 1 teaspoon turmeric powder
- ½ teaspoon grated ginger
- 1 teaspoon honey (optional)
- Lemon slice for garnish

Instructions:

1. In a small saucepan, bring the water to a boil.
2. Add the turmeric powder and grated ginger to the boiling water.
3. Reduce the heat and let the mixture simmer for 5 minutes to infuse the flavors.
4. Remove from heat and strain the tea into a mug.
5. If desired, add honey to sweeten.
6. Garnish with a lemon slice.
7. Sip the warm and soothing turmeric ginger tea for its potential anti-inflammatory properties and refreshing taste.

Serving: 1 serving

Preparation time: 10 minutes

Nutritional Information per Serving: Calories: 10, Protein: 0g, Fat: 0g, Carbohydrates: 3g, Fiber: 0g

Sparkling Water with Citrus Slices

- 2 cups sparkling water
- Slices of citrus fruits (such as lemon, lime, and orange)
- Ice cubes

Instructions:

1. Fill a glass with ice cubes.
2. Add slices of citrus fruits to the glass.

3. Pour sparkling water over the citrus slices and ice cubes.
4. Stir gently to combine.
5. Sip the refreshing sparkling water with citrus slices as a hydrating and flavorful beverage.

Serving: 1 serving

Preparation time: 5 minutes

Nutritional Information per Serving: Calories: 0, Protein: 0g, Fat: 0g, Carbohydrates: 0g, Fiber: 0g

Conclusion

The mouthwatering array of recipes in The Osteoporosis Diet Cookbook is created to energize your system and support strong, healthy bones. This cookbook offers a variety of filling meals and snacks that are good for bone health, with an emphasis on nutrient-rich foods and delectable tastes.

We've looked at a range of delectable foods throughout the book, from filling breakfast alternatives to wholesome lunches, tantalizing dinners, healthy snacks, and energizing drinks. The elements in each mix have been carefully chosen to support bone strength and general health.

You may actively prevent osteoporosis and maintain ideal bone health by including these recipes in your daily practice. You also can control your food consumption thanks to the nutritional details offered for each dish.

Keep in mind that taste and diversity are not sacrificed when eating a diet that is great for your bones. Eating for bone health, according to the Osteoporosis Diet Cookbook, maybe a joyful and enjoyable activity. So don your apron and head to the kitchen to start a gastronomic adventure that will boost your general vitality and fortify your bones.

Future meals will be scrumptious and healthy for the bones! Make sure to drop a review if you enjoyed this book

www.ingramcontent.com/pod-product-compliance
Lightning Source LLC
Chambersburg PA
CBHW072251260726
48657CB00006BA/2369